SEVEN BILLION
CURES FOR CANCER

SEVEN BILLION CURES FOR CANCER

AND YOU ARE ONE OF THEM

FRANK RUANE

MOUNTAIN ARBOR
PRESS

MOUNTAIN ARBOR
PRESS
Alpharetta, GA

The opinions expressed in this book are those of the author and are based upon information and data obtained at the time of publication. Opinions in this book are provided for information purposes only and are not intended as a substitute for the medical advice of a competent and knowledgeable physician. The reader should always consult a trusted physician in matters relating to his/her health and particularly with respect to any condition that may require immediate medical attention. The information provided in this book should not be construed as personal medical advice or instruction. Self-diagnosis and self-treatment are not recommended and may indeed be dangerous. Readers who fail to consult competent, trusted physicians assume the risk of any injuries or illness.

ISBN: 978-1-63183-741-8 - Paperback
eISBN: 978-1-63183-742-5 - ePub
eISBN: 978-1-63183-743-2 - mobi

Printed in the United States of America   0 2 2 4 2 0

⊗This paper meets the requirements of ANSI/NISO Z39.48-1992 (Permanence of Paper)

Protocel® is a registered trademark of PMB Technologies, LLC, Dover, Delaware (2002).

Glucovance® is a registered trademark of Merck Sante, SAS, Lyon, France (2000).

For Jennifer,
the love of my life,
the thrill of a lifetime

Thank you,
Laura and Maria,
for always being there.

I DIDN'T KNOW

When I used to pick your things up off the floor,
I didn't know I would one day kneel in tears
Clutching something because it smelled like you.
When I couldn't find time to listen to you,
I didn't know I would one day give anything
To hear your voice or hear you call my name again.

When I left without kissing you goodbye,
I didn't know I would one day lose my breath
At the thought of never kissing you again.
When I was too busy with other things,
I didn't know I would one day fall prey
To the unbearable silence you left behind . . .

And for those times I failed to say I love you,
I am, in the quiet of my darkened room,
Asking God to tell you
That I will love you with all my heart
Until my last breath on my last day.

February 2019

CONTENTS

INTRODUCTION

*There are two ways to be fooled. One is to believe
what is not true; the other is to refuse to believe
what is true.*

—Soren Kierkegaard

This may well be one of the shortest self-help books
ever. They used to have condensed versions of classic
novels that you could purchase in the drugstore. These
shortcuts got many of us through book reports in high
school. They covered all the important parts without all
the boring details. That's what I've tried to do here. I've
read all the excellent books on self-healing cancer, and I
believe people who are seriously ill, or are caring for
someone who is seriously ill, don't want to read about the
mechanics of cell biology and technical research data.
They (we) want to know what's wrong and what do I do
about it. This is a shortcut version of the cancer novel that,
I believe, brings you the best input from some of the finest
scientific and research minds in the world. I've given
several references to books and websites if you want to
read about blood chemistry and cell biology, but, I'm
guessing, right now isn't the time. So, consider this home
base. I've separated the chaff from the grain. Consider it

the resource that starts you thinking on your own and reaching out to the vast amounts of help available.

All books, all papers, and all studies are slanted toward an opinion. This is mine. It's just my side of the story based upon what I saw and experienced, and I have used the data I have uncovered to support my beliefs. There may be conflicting data and varying opinions, but the base philosophy of this work is true and accurate. It's a philosophy for which there is no logical dispute; that is, we have viable, proven, successful alternatives to Big Cancer Care. If you disagree with me, you have to disagree with the brilliant scientists and researchers who have laid the foundation, often at personal risk, for a monumental change in how we view medicine.

There are approximately seven billion people on our planet, and we were all Divinely created with the ability to heal ourselves. In fact, the average adult may have cured him or herself of cancer several times without knowing it. If we are healthy, it happens when we sleep. That means we have no conscious control over it. It's automatic, like heartbeat and breathing. If we are not healthy, we need extra help. This is where nutrition and attitude come in. We are a complete package. We are not physical beings with a spirit; we are spiritual beings with a body. There are seven billion cures for cancer on the planet, and you are one of them.

CHAPTER ONE

THE WAKE-UP CALL

Once you eliminate the impossible, whatever remains, no matter how improbable, must be the truth.

—Sir Arthur Conan Doyle

THE BEGINNING

Cancer treatment used to be wards in local hospitals doing the best they could to treat the disease. Then, while no one was looking, cancer treatment centers reared their greedy little heads and turned into the medical version of the oil industry, with multi-building centers and specialty areas. It's even Big Business for private practices. Unfortunately, medicine can't cure cancer. Food and exercise can't cure cancer. Fasting and chemotherapy can't cure cancer, and surgery can't cure cancer. In the whole wide world, there is one thing, and only one thing, that can totally cure cancer: your body. **Do not let your diagnosis determine how you are going to live your life.**

The body is an amazing machine that requires

maintenance and occasional repairs. Most repairs are a result of a lack of maintenance. Yes, it's true, there are those issues that you can inherit, but most are caused by outside influences like food additives and chemicals. The important thing to remember is that healing is done from the inside out, not from the outside in. Mainstream medical is learning this and is gradually incorporating holistic and alternative approaches in combination with those that pay for the golf cart and the beach house. Even if a patient goes the whole nine yards of conventional treatment, it's still mandatory to give the body the support it needs to handle the abuse.

SUPPORT OR NO SUPPORT

It didn't take long before I realized that my wife's treatment wasn't going to feed the bulldog. I made the decision that additional help was necessary. When you reach this point, and you will, it is helpful to have outside support from family members and friends. I had the support of amazing family and friends, most especially two incredible sisters-in-law and three sons. On the downside, however, very few people supported me in my quest to reduce, or eliminate, the amount of Big Business medical care and add natural support. If you choose to boycott mainstream approaches, you may find resistance, even from the most supportive. You will need the strength of conviction and knowledge to bring a strong argument to the table.

CONDITIONING

Okay, why the resistance to alternative treatments from otherwise supportive people? Actually, a few reasons. First, it's a comfort zone. It's easy just to follow what everyone else is doing even if it's wrong, and especially when we're afraid. Secondly, it's like a multiple-choice exam. When we don't know the answer, we go with what feels most right and keep our fingers crossed. Additionally, we have a fear of being different. However, we still have to deal with the very real possibility that everyone else may be wrong. It is, by definition, a rock and a hard place.

SO WHY THE BOOK?

In February of 2018, my wife was diagnosed with Stage IIIA lung cancer. Her name was Jennifer, and she was the love of my life and my soul mate. Although we didn't know it at the time, it had metastasized to her opposite shoulder and neck. Over the next few months, there were hints that there may be another way to deal with this than traditional medicine. What kept gnawing at me was that her treatment was too quick, too formulated, too businesslike, and too conveyor belt. Our caregivers didn't know our fears or hopes or questions or our situation, and didn't seem like they wanted to. It was so department store, it was creepy. To them we were a tumor, a very lucrative one at that.

We had little or no opportunity to ask questions, and our request for additional, nontraditional testing was ignored.

Additionally, there wasn't any time to do any research or make any informed decisions, and we were not encouraged to. Any questions we were asked were only so they had enough information to prescribe more medication. Could this be the exception to the rule? Sure. But the important thing is it happened, and if it happened to us, it's happening to others elsewhere around the country. The most caring, efficient, loving cancer-treatment centers in the country still need to make a profit to stay in business.

THE TITLE SAYS IT ALL!

When was the last time you heard of total chemical treatments curing cancer? You hear of advances and you hear of progress and you hear of hope for this thing and that thing, and sometimes people live longer than the five-year mark. That's nice. If you have been listening at all over the past ten years or so, you will notice you keep hearing the word "immune" pop up. Wonder why? Well, it's because they are learning that the most successful protocols involve stimulating the immune system in some way. They have come to realize that it's the immune system that is responsible for the cure, and the more successful approaches incorporate it. Not only that, they advertise it like it's a new concept. Then again, I guess it is if you consider the idea has only been around since we started learning to walk upright as a species.

Well, there has been an immune system booster for a long time. You may have heard of it. It's called food, or more precisely, nutrition. It's been in all the papers. The downside to it is that we have continually reduced food's effectiveness over the decades with genetic engineering, adding pesticides and growth hormones, so we have to invent chemicals to do what food used to do. Fortunately for us, we have chemicals to reduce the effect of the chemicals. Cheery thought.

There was an advertisement on TV many years ago that, I believe, involved smoking. The announcer was talking down to the audience like a small child because, he said, when I speak to you like adults, you don't listen. So, the seven-billion-dollar question would be, "Why not just use natural immune boosters that don't kill you?" The seven-billion-dollar answer would be because you can't patent it or make money off of it, which is, first and foremost, the primary consideration.

WHY NOT ASK WHY?

Thirty or forty years ago, what a doctor told you wasn't questioned. That was back in the day of exploratory and needless operations. Today, we have too much information, and it's too easy to find. Not only that, it's reliable. So why are so many people getting cancer? Primarily, lifestyle. The food we eat and the water we drink are systemically executing us. Then we get diagnosed, and without a second thought, we throw ourselves at the cancer interests and the radiation guy and the dietitian and so on. We act like sheep and take no responsibility for our own health.

I'm not telling you what to do. I am, however, suggesting that if you get herded into the chemo lineup, it should be because you have done a lot of research and believe it is the right thing for you.

Cancer Is Not an Emergency!

Your first reaction is going to be, *What do I do now? Where do I start?* Well, the first thing you do is nothing. STOP! If you are too afraid to stop the wheels of pressure, then at least back off long enough to think. Unless you have a bodily function that has stopped working, cancer is not an emergency. It took years for your tumor to develop, and it's not going to change in a week no matter how aggressive they say it is. Ask for additional tests, look for second opinions, and get as much information on integrative and alternative treatments you can find. You have time to look at all your options and decide what would be the best course of treatment for you. They will tell you, like they told us, "If you don't start right now, you won't survive." Okay, you may not survive. But starting treatment a week or two later won't make a difference. Don't be driven by fear. Manage the situation, don't let it, or them, manage you. Even "aggressive" cancers aren't aggressive until they start treating and feeding it.

Find out if your oncologist will support nontraditional approaches, or get one who will. Look at every alternate option out there. "Not all cancers are the same." This is one of the areas where traditional medicine quotes are correct. When you ask about cure rates, this is the phrase they are taught to say that is pretty much a catchall that lets the fish off the hook. Before you begin a program, make sure you have looked at all options. Read, read, read.

THE ELEPHANT IN THE ROOM

If there is a discussion in this text that could set the tempo for it all, it would be this. In fact, if you don't read any further, your life should, in some way, change. They call it "wag the dog." Simply put, it is a means of preventing you from focusing on one area while your attention is diverted to another. A good example would be global warming. I'm not saying global warming isn't a problem, because I don't know, but we have bigger fish to fry.

In retrospect, we are poisoning our bodies beyond repair with pesticides, genetically modified foods, over-the-counter drugs, prescription medications, laundry chemicals, cosmetics lotions and soaps, antibiotics, and electronics. The hard reality is that it is difficult not to come in contact with harmful substances many times each day, especially carcinogens.

Many surgeries are unnecessary and many can be avoided, especially cardiac. Radiation from scans causes cancer, and for some reason, we try to prevent fevers, one of the greatest tools we have for killing viruses. Additionally, through the work of the brilliant and courageous Dr. Andrew Wakefield, we know that even vaccines are dangerous and can cause childhood abnormalities and autism. These vaccines are around mainly because of pressure from pharmaceuticals. Sadly, since a bill signed by President Reagan in the 1980s, manufacturers of vaccines are "immune from prosecution" for any harm they cause.

Global warming? Okay, I'll bite. But, until we notice the elephant and we are willing to look at the truth, we will continue to have no way out of the hopper. There are seven billion of us, and we are each unique and special. We are each in sole possession of the most magnificent, self-healing, self-regulating machine in the history of the universe: the human body.

> *It's easier to fool people than to convince them they have been fooled.*
>
> —Mark Twain

When the unthinkable happens and we are diagnosed with a serious illness, there are three reasons we don't look at more than one option for a cure: fear, ignorance, and conditioning. Since we were small, we have been conditioned to go to the doctor with every sniffle and to accept antibiotics as though they are routine and safe and to never question the doctor and to always throw our well-being totally into the hands of the professionals. When it comes to our health, we've become a nation of sheep with a knee-jerk reaction to illness, because it's easy, it's routine, and we don't have to think about it. It's comforting to be led around by a medical nose ring. It's stupid and dangerous . . . but comforting.

It's only been since the internet, and the information

highway, that most of us have given any thought to alternatives or taking any control over our health. Reflex medicine is a habit and a hard one to break, but we need to learn to trust ourselves and take control. The irony of the whole thing is that the people who are most guilty of reflex medicine and never straying from the traditional are the healthcare professionals themselves.

THE MEDS JOKE

If it sounds like I'm being disrespectful, I am. But now, let me ask you a couple of questions. Do you know that Americans are the most overmedicated people in the history of civilization? Are you one of the four people in the world who can listen to the advertisements and still think prescription drugs are safe?

It's assumed we're all on some form of medication. And we are. If you are an adult in the United States and not on some prescription medication, you are one of 16 percent of the population. Does anyone beside me find that strange, or even a little scary? We are all on medication of some sort for some reason. Every third advertisement on TV is an ad for some drug, and the side effects take as long to say as the ad. It's epidemic proportions, and the drugs are too easy to get, and they are all harmful. Even the ones that should be fairly innocuous, like cold medications, are dangerous. Prescription drugs are kept off the list of killers because, if they were, they would be ahead of heart attacks, cancer, automobile accidents, and gunshot wounds. 'Nuff said.

ACCUMULATING POISONS

Jennifer was constantly sick or had digestive problems and constantly kept a small bucket close by. Additionally, she was listless, had little strength, and had difficulty managing even the smallest of tasks. The problem was that it was during a period of time where she should have been over the effects of chemo and on the road to recovery. Sure, the cancer was still there, but it was not at a stage that would have given her that much varied discomfort. Something wasn't right.

IT WAS A CHEMICAL FREE-FOR-ALL

One evening, I happened to glance at the pill-bottle basket. I took eleven bottles of Jennifer's pills and put them on the dining room table. I went online and began looking at what they were, what they did, and what were the most common side effects. What I found was disheartening. These may have been killing her faster than the cancer. Some of the drugs were to combat the effects of other drugs. Three of them were to combat the effects of the chemo poison. Two of them were fighting against two of the others, and so on. Think about it. If you've been ingesting sixteen bottles of pills, these pills are compounds of several other chemicals. So, it's logical to assume you could have eighty or more different chemicals. What does the body do with this information?

To complicate matters even more, this was all while she

was wearing a painkiller patch 24/7. The total of the most common side effects added up to thirty-two, in all, with no duplicates. There was everything from dizziness to loss of appetite to blurred vision to back pain, and the list goes on. No wonder she was sick all the time. By the way, "When you see a woman with no hair and a bandana on her head, you are not looking at a cancer patient—you're looking at a chemotherapy patient" (Chris Wark).

THE FUNNEL

This is what I call the integrated system, or cattle prod, that forces you into the mainstream medical system, and there are no windows to the outside. The insurance companies don't recognize viable alternatives to poison and drugs. Medical students are discouraged from thinking past drugs. Oncologists scoff at nontraditional testing, and important alternative data are not included in any mainstream publications. All the while, Big Pharma is raising the ponies for the show.

Remember that modern medicine is reactive, not proactive. Let me repeat that in case you're reading fast: Big Medicine is reactive, not proactive. Let's take obesity, for example. There is no money in preventing it. The money comes in a myriad of gimmicks, drugs, and surgeries to treat and sustain it rather than convincing you that you need a lifestyle change. Even diets make money. If you want to call it a disease, fine, but if you had any disease that could be cured by just changing your lifestyle, wouldn't you be foolish not to do it? Well, that's the way it is with most of today's ailments.

PRESCRIPTION DRUGS

All prescription drugs have side effects. Some are more dangerous than others, and some are lethal. The risks of prescription drugs are what they call actuarial. That means their distribution is subject to actuarial tables that measure the risks compared to the advantages. If a certain margin between the two exists, the drug is given the green light for the general public. It is not uncommon for a drug to help a particular condition in 60 percent of cases and have eight or ten major side effects. Listen closely to the advertisements. Some prescription drugs have been shown to cause cancer and other serious ailments, and the human body can't withstand the barrage of all the chemicals for long. Eventually, the body's defense mechanisms will become saturated and will give up. Unfortunately, and it's sad, but the consideration is frequently the lesser of two evils. It's not my intent to step on toes, but it's not my fault if you have big feet.

THE RIPPLE EFFECT

Let's say, for example, you are taking a drug to control psoriasis. To begin with, the drug has an almost 0 percent chance of actually curing the disease, and about a 60 percent chance of controlling it. Remember, if they cure the disease, you are off the payroll. Okay, that's fair enough if that gives you the comfort level you're looking for.

So, where's the problem? Well, it's called the ripple effect, and it's why they list side effects when they advertise drugs on TV. Fortunately, most side effects are short term and temporary, but many are not. The patient is basically making decisions between rocks and hard places and evaluating their quality of life.

So, on one hand, the drug is controlling the psoriasis, but on the other hand, it is sending toxins to your liver that, after a time, the liver can no longer filter. Also, the synthetic elements that the body doesn't recognize get passed through, for the most part, but others get stored somewhere until the body knows what to do with them. It's almost like it's putting them on a shelf so your immune system can study them.

The residual effects can affect not only the liver but the kidneys, the spleen, and any of the vital organs that filter the blood or impurities. If you are taking drugs that require you to have liver function tests periodically, weigh that against the benefits. It's not rocket surgery.

START HERE

If you do continue reading and you only remember a handful of thoughts I've presented here, let the following be one of them: If you took a perfectly healthy adult and put them on the cancer-treatment medication that Jennifer was given, they would probably not survive. You may live a little longer, but so what. If Hippocrates were alive today, he would no doubt wonder how the human body can fight both the cancer and the cure. This is one of the issues that got me started on my quest to find a better way.

They give you drugs to halt the spread of the cancer that make you nauseous. Then drugs to stop the nausea that give you diarrhea, then drugs to stop the diarrhea, then drugs to stop the constipation the anti-diarrhea drugs give you, but they make your mouth dry and make you dizzy so they give you drugs to stop that and on and on and on. Good grief! Has anyone besides me wondered why we don't invest in cancer-treatment centers on Wall Street? It's a booming business, and it's not going anywhere. It won't have a downturn because it doesn't depend on the economy. Do we need all the pieces of this puzzle to see what the picture is?

ANOTHER ATTENTION-GETTER

Sitting in a chemo ward is one of the most chilling experiences you can imagine. Jennifer was there with about twenty-five other people in a line of chairs in an area that was originally designed for twelve. No one really understands what's going on, and you can tell by the looks on their faces no one has any idea there is anything else out there. It was that way with us also, at first. The really sad part is that if you took a room of one hundred cancer patients on chemo and asked how many are reviewing alternative or supplemental treatments, probably no hands would go up. That pretty much sums up the reason for this book.

During our second round is when Jennifer got her diet briefing. It took about ten minutes, and she was given a bound packet that looked more like they were selling time-shares. It was an expensive-looking kit, suitable for the conference table in any boardroom. I have to wonder if the chemo chair is a good place to give a diet lecture, but that's just me. As she was sitting there, people in hazmat suits were injecting nuclear waste into her bloodstream that would have her urinating salsa for the next seven days. Then they wanted her to pay attention to their recipe for cookies or something. As good a time as any, I guess.

DON'T ASK QUESTIONS? WHY NOT?

I wanted to know Jennifer's chances of survival. What were we up against? Would they call it a long shot at the track? Throughout the course of her treatment, I asked about survival statistics. There is evidently no real answer. It's like giving an interview to reporters. They told me, "Well, there's all kinds of cancer," or "Only your physician would have that information." Okay, we've established that, but what about our kind? It was apparent no one wanted to think that hard. If you asked a pro quarterback how many games he won last year, he could say, "Well, it depends on what you mean by win," or "Sometimes we came in second, and that's sort of a win, in a sense" (compared to third, I guess). Or, how about "I don't know, only Coach would have that information." This is what we had to deal with for a year. (This is where I should insert the emoji with the crossed eyes and hanging tongue.)

THE IMPETUS TO KEEP GOING

As I have mentioned, there were signals and occurrences that called my attention to the fact that there were things the medical community either didn't know or refused to look into. After a time, I realized it was actually a combination. I had no medical knowledge, and the cancer scare was new to me. Throughout the process of trying to save Jennifer, I relied heavily on my instinct and intuition. This is mentioned later in this work. Something was wrong. Something didn't feel right, and I started reading and reading every night and on weekends and every chance I got for months.

I have the utmost respect for the medical community. In time, however, I realized that there is a world of information out there that is valuable and healing and exciting to read about that's just not crossing the street to the cancer store. My guess is that it will not happen until we can separate the desire to heal from the desire to grow a business.

> *All things being equal, the simplest explanation tends to be the right one.*
>
> —Occam's Razor (William of Ockham)

THE LONG-TERM MEDS INSANITY

One of the reasons I wrote this book is because I heard rumors about mainstream cancer treatments, but took them with a grain of salt. Now, I was seeing it with my own eyes. In the introduction of this work, I mention that one of the two ways to be fooled is to not believe something that is true. As Jennifer's health began to deteriorate, she began to develop other ailments. On one occasion, I had to take her to the emergency room because I could no longer control her pain adequately. During the examination, they discovered she had gone into arteria fibrillation, or AFib for short. Simply put, this is where the heart beats very rapidly and increases the risk of stroke. They put her in intensive care to begin treatment, which included dangerous beta blockers, without knowing for sure what caused it in an otherwise cardio-healthy woman.

This is not anecdotal or a rumor passed down by family members. They looked me in the eye and told me they had no idea what was causing it. Really? They offered the possibility of a combination of things. Hell, I could have told you that. For sure it was a combination of things. Maybe being on twenty-one different medications in thirteen months had something to do with it. Think? Why not try to eliminate or reduce the risk? Then again, let's not confuse the issue with logic.

After a couple of days of liquid meds, the cardiologist met me in the hall outside her room to tell me he put her on a beta blocker to continue her treatment when she got

Frank Ruane

home. When I asked how long she would be on them, he responded with, "Until she can't tolerate them anymore." I thought to myself, *I can't believe it, they're writing my script for me.* When they put you on this stuff, they totally ignore the tremendous damage it is doing to you and have no plan to get you off of it. This needs to change. Demand a plan to get off of it. Find out what you need to do, and do it.

> *Only dead fish go with the flow.*
>
> —Unknown

CHAPTER TWO

THE NEED FOR CHANGE

It takes less courage to stand up and speak than to sit and listen.

—Sir Winston Churchill

WHERE TO BEGIN?

In the first four or five nights of study, I had learned what I believed was enough to help Jennifer through the crisis, even if it was just to complement Big Medicine for now. Big Medicine can scoff if they want to, but the people who question their methods are not snake oil salesmen or charlatans. Many of these visionaries are physicians and surgeons and PhD biochemists and physicists who have had the courage to come forward and buck established medicine, the one-trick pony. The hard part was getting Jennifer to adhere to it. Really hard. In fact, it didn't happen.

THE QUESTION OF THE CENTURY: SUGAR, NO SUGAR?

Before we say anything about the sugar controversy, it is important to understand that, although it is true cancer cells have a voracious appetite for sugar, they also have the ability to feed on fat and glutamine. This is why it is so important to do the additional testing. Your protocol may require multiple compounds to fight, or block, all paths of nutrition for your particular type of cancer. Melanomas, for example, thrive on fat, and other types may thrive on something else. However, all have appetites for sugar about eighteen times faster than normal cells.

Robert Lustig, MD, through the University of California TV, explains that the two most opposite diets, Atkins and Japanese, have something very important in common: the Atkins diet is all fat and no carbs, and the Japanese diet is all carbs and no fat. However, in spite of their base differences, they both eliminate fructose or sugar.

Jane McLelland published a work that looks at the success of off-label (cheap) drugs to solve the problem of multiple nutrition paths for cancer cells. In her work, she notes the importance of staying away from high-dose chemo and the importance of attacking the problem from different directions and understanding the sad realization that stem cells will be left behind to cause havoc. For some reason, they ignore this little tidbit of information when they put you on chemo. No biggie.

Cancer cells have the ability to divide uncontrollably

and generate hordes of new tumor cells. Much of the energy they consume is sugar. There is another side to the coin, however, and that is if you starve cancer cells of their glucose, they will find another fuel source or find another way to get glucose. Another study, a Belgium study, was the result of a nine-year study that ended in 2017. It suggests that sugar produces more cancer-causing genes, known as Ras proteins, that fuel aggressive tumors.

Additionally, a recent MIT study, under Matthew Vander Heiden, MD, PhD, after studying the Warburg effect found that amino acids contribute to the carbon atoms found in the cell and comprise most of the mass. He concluded it's not just the Warburg effect, but more importantly, how does glucose-to-lactate conversion help cells use amino acids and therefore build more cells?

> *If I won an award for laziness, I'd send someone to pick it up for me.*
>
> —Unknown

THE BOTTOM LINE

Regardless of which side of the coin you fall on, the fact remains that many people cure themselves of cancer each year, and they do it by limiting sugar intake, following an organic greens diet, and avoiding animal fats.

Let me quote Mary Jo Parker, nutritionist, who cured herself of metastasized cancer and is author of the book of the same name: "If you cannot maintain a normal blood sucrose level, you have a zero percent chance of beating metastasized cancer."

> *If you take your medicine, you will get better in four days. If you don't take your medicine, you will get better in five, without the side effects.*
>
> —Unknown

First Things First: Dispelling the Myths

Most clinical studies have varying or even conflicting points of view. With the exception of the American Cancer Society, many myths have been brought to light by the world scientific community:

- **Chemo kills CTCs (circulating tumor cells).** No. Only the body can cure on the quantum level. That means that if you live long enough, the cancer will come back with an appetite that can feed freely on whatever it wants in the absence of your immune system.
- **Chemo kills stem cells.** Actually, no it doesn't. Stem cells are new cells that, to simplify, have not received an assignment yet, like becoming a hair follicle or a foot or an internal organ. This is why stem-cell therapy is such a big deal. Some cells will remain in a non-dividing state until

activated by a disease. These are adult stem cells. The purer forms are the embryo cells that are easily motivated, and therefore the subject of much controversial research.

- **The sun causes skin cancer.** No, not true. We have been in the sun all day for 5,950 years, and now, all of a sudden, in the last half of the twentieth century, we're getting skin cancer. The truth is that the chemicals in our environment and in our food and in our water are radically changing the way our bodies process everything, including the energy from the sun.

- **A lot of cancer is hereditary.** Not necessarily. Having the same gene as a parent does not necessarily mean it's hereditary. "So, if my grandfather and father both had heart disease, I will probably get it too." It is probably true that you are predisposed to heart disease if you choose the same destructive lifestyle choices. If you have the habit of eating ham hocks and lard every morning, then you are placing yourself at the same risk for heart disease. Then you ask, "What about the gene they found in me?" Good for you. It has to be encouraged to surface.

- **It's still your lifestyle that allows those genes to emerge.** True. Your parents and grandparents probably had the same one. Your immune system can easily keep them suppressed and is probably doing it right now. If you radically change your diet from that of your parents, or grandparents, you will radically reduce your chances of developing the same diseases.

- **If we don't get started right now, today, you won't survive.** Not true. That's what they told Jennifer. The truth is that you probably have time. Your tumor did not appear overnight. As John McDougall, MD, said, an average breast cancer tumor may have been growing for seven to twelve years before it could be felt. Again, unless it is stopping a bodily function, cancer is not an emergency.

- **You have a better chance of survival if detected early.** No. As I will explain later, according to John McDougall, MD, early detection is, well, misleading. Early or late, the treatment course you take decides your chances of recovery. In fact, recent developments in prostate cancer suggest we should not jump into treatment right away. Prostate cancer is one of the slowest growing, and it may take years to notice a change after a positive PSA is found (PSA stands for prostate-specific antigen test and attempts to give the degree of probability of developing prostate cancer). It is now believed that men are rushed into radical treatments for prostate cancer long before it is necessary.

- **Chemo cures cancer.** (If I had access to emoji right now, this is where I would insert the one with the crossed eyes and tongue hanging out again.) Well, no, actually chemo doesn't cure cancer. It temporarily suppresses it. I know a statement like that is very controversial, so I'm glad it wasn't me who came up with it. Many brilliant professionals are saying it. Chemotherapy actually doesn't "cure" cancer. Sure, Uncle Harvey had chemo fifteen years ago and is still going strong. Okay, I get it. Then again, I was in Reno in 2003 when a patron near me won a small car on the slot machines. Did it make me want to turn my mortgage into eight hundred pounds of quarters and slot my life away? Uh . . . no.

The brain works every day: seven days a week, three hundred sixty-five days each year, from the day we are born until the day we fall in love.

—Unknown

OKAY, WHAT DOES CHEMO DO?

If chemotherapy doesn't cure cancer, then what does it do? Well, for starters, it sterilizes you like you spent three minutes in the microwave or got dental x-rays every day for a year. Chemo beats the tumor into submission so it becomes too small to see. It reduces the size of the active cells, but not the stem cells. They call that dormant, or being in remission. However, it's still circulating in your blood like a troll under a bridge in the form of CTCs, or circulating tumor cells, unaffected by the chemo.

Big Medicine needs the gold star to put in the cure column, and five years was the success-rate turning point. Convenient? Yes, I know. Actually, there were people cured by Dr. Johanna Budwig, and in ninety days. Dr. Budwig is the PhD physicist and physician who created the Budwig Protocol, a diet which has been credited for curing cancer for more than forty years. But who's counting? Statistically, if you die at five years and a day, it is still considered a cure. However, the cancer is, as I mentioned earlier, always there and will come back with a vengeance unless a good dietary protocol lets your body cure it. Are there instances where the cancer does not come back after chemo and surgery? Absolutely yes. Would you want to take those odds to the roulette table?

> *I'm old, so my remaining chance for a smoking hot body is cremation.*
>
> —Unknown

IT'S NOT ALL DIET

No, it's not all diet, but that's most of it. You hear it over and over again: you are what you eat. There are, in fact, hundreds of people refusing the poison of chemotherapy and healing themselves of cancer with diet. It's not a myth. It's very real and very encouraging. It is important that this work not be all the information you receive on healing yourself, but rather a catalyst to encourage you to keep on searching.

Many of us are calorie challenged and are enjoying a larger portion of the real me. On the other hand, you may be just someone who needs to push away from the table about one muffin sooner. Whatever your situation, it's important to understand that something encouraged your body to grow tumors. Eliminate that outside stimulus, and the body will eliminate the tumors. Biochemistry 101.

Don't wait for the storm to pass. Dance in the rain.

—Unknown

A SCARY TRUTH

Since 1950, advances in diet, disease prevention, hygiene, and the way we can strengthen our immune system and enhance our overall health have not changed the way medicine treats our ailments. What does that mean? It means that modern medicine treats the same way it did in the middle of the twentieth century. Is that encouraging or what? It treats by after-the-fact reaction to disease and treating symptoms, rather than with alternate education, prevention, and alternative lifestyle, which by the way, society is ready for and craving.

Is My Treatment Curative or Palliative?

Okay, you've been given a course of treatment. Ask your doctor which one it is. You may be one of those lucky few who are being given a curative course of treatment, where the final outcome is expected to be a cure with only a marginal chance of returning. Unfortunately, most are not.

Most are palliative, which means they are trying to extend a life by two or three years, or get you to the five-year mark so you can go in the win column. In a large room full of people, ask how many know of someone who has had cancer, and how many do they know of who have been completely cured. It could be an eye-opener.

I find it hard to understand why many people don't know which treatment straw they have drawn. At the time of this writing, Jennifer, for example, is expecting a cure, even though she is undergoing a palliative approach, where they are looking for three years before trying a new approach.

Basically, this means she will continue to have a life of unalienable misery and pain for whatever time she has left. And I can tell you, misery like that isn't cheap. At the risk of sounding repetitive, with chemo you have about a 51 percent chance of living three years, and if you do nothing, you have a 49 percent chance. However, that's doing nothing, with no special nutritional support. If you find that hard to understand, don't bet on sports.

DRUGS AND DATA

The nice people who bring you the drugs also bring the data that support using them. Thank you for not forcing us to think. Oh, and they also publish the results. Hmmm, sounds like a marriage made in heaven. The drug companies send sales reps into the physician's offices to push the latest concoction. Oh! I almost forgot; they provide the literature that gives the clinical data on what can happen to you if you take it for too long without a break. If you ask most physicians, and they are honest, they will tell you they don't have the time to do their own research and so they rely on the data they are provided by the nice lady in the business suit who brings the shrimp cocktails and champagne at lunch. Is that nice or what?

Do some chemotherapy drugs cause cancer? In a word, yes. Will they tell you that? Only if you ask, and only if they have been told. It's not only the carcinogenic chemicals, but the radiation from PET scans and CT scans is equivalent to numerous standard x-rays. Every day, I watch Jennifer desperately struggling to survive the cure, and it not only gets me up several times a night, but it breaks my heart.

CHAPTER THREE

INSIDE BIG-BUSINESS MEDICINE

Sunshine is the first medicine you will take each day. A day without sunshine is like, well . . . night.

—Unknown

ACT TWO AND THE TWO BIGGEST MISUNDERSTANDINGS

The check is in the mail and we got it all. Maybe the check is in the mail and maybe it's not, but the only things they got with your surgery were what could be seen and your cancelled check. It's a process where they cut until the testing doesn't show cancer cells anymore. It's a good start, but unfortunately, the damage is on the quantum level. It's in the cells circulating throughout your body. Other diseases run unhindered and rampant. What good is it if the medical community calls you cancer-free, but you suffer from every disease under the sun and die from some common virus that a healthy immune system would have destroyed? Reasonable question, no?

THE BIRTH OF BABY CHEMO

Chemotherapy originated in the WWII years when researchers did autopsies on soldiers who died from exposure to mustard gas and found there were toxic changes in bone marrow that developed into cells. Then the lightbulb went off and a nitrogen mustard compound was developed that showed promise against lymphoma. This actually served as a model for many years and led to the alkylating agents (does this word ring a bell, or is it me?). Mustard gas is actually mentioned in the diet guide that we were given by the chemo center. You can't make this stuff up.

THE IMPORTANCE OF ADDITIONAL TESTS

We have already established that not all cancers are the same. Even if you are using a totally natural protocol, your particular type of cancer will respond to some things and not respond to others. This is true for both natural and synthetic treatments.

Oncologists take the road of tradition and follow the guidelines recommended by NCCN (National Comprehensive Cancer Network). I don't recall our oncologist telling us what tests they used to determine the course of treatment for Jennifer. They looked for a marker that she did not have, but decided to go with the immunotherapy course in addition to chemo. A marker is a characteristic of a tumor cell that makes it more vulnerable to immunotherapy. In all fairness to these good people, however, ambulance chasers follow them everywhere, and I don't blame them for an ounce of caution.

I gave our oncology nurse a letter of request for an RGCC test. This very accurate test was originally used in Greece and is sometimes still called the Greek test. Now, it is completed in several areas of the country and is actually not that expensive. I don't know if the insurance companies will pay for it, but I'd take up a collection if I could get it for Jennifer. Additionally, I provided our oncology nurse a ten-page report supporting the benefits of the RGCC test, and I requested she ask our doctor if we could get one.

She said she'd never heard of it and, after scoffing at me, said she would relay that request. We never heard back. What our oncology liaison failed to realize was that I was not trying to step on anyone's toes or interfere with their course of treatment. I was a husband willing to do anything to save his wife. Why doesn't this compute?

WHAT THE RGCC DOES

The beauty of the RGCC, or the Greek, test is that it identifies the specific characteristics of the cells and identifies substances, natural and chemo, that will destroy it. Seems like it's worth a shot to me. The truth is that the RGCC Group detects early stages of cancer and helps monitor existing cancers. Additionally, it is said to give valuable information on which chemo drugs and which natural substances will attack the individual cells. Those who scoff at the out-of-club testing say it's only about 60 percent accurate. Surely you jest. If traditional cancer treatment were 60 percent effective, they'd be world heroes.

All suggested treatments have skeptics, and it's actually a good thing. It keeps people honest. The RGCC has several different testing stages. The tests include a series, which allows you to check and follow malignant cell count: the OncoTRACE, which provides information about the presence of CTCs, and others that give viable information about the characteristics of the individual cells and what they will respond to or not respond to. If it's not 100 percent accurate, then what good is it? It's still not snake oil, and the odds are it will offer some valuable insight that could keep you out of the hospital from a reaction.

Another very valuable test is the ONCOblot (Ecto-Nicotinamide Adenine Dinucleotide Oxidase Disulfide-Thiol Exchanger 2, or ENOX2 for short). This is a test developed for early detection of very small amounts of cancer regardless of where it is in the body. It can detect as little as two million cancer cells, which is a tumor the size of the head of a pin, in as many as twenty-five different cancers. Even if its value is highly exaggerated, it's still a hundred times better than having bagel-sized tumors cut out. Think about it—it detects Stage 0 cancer. This means that if it is detected by the ONCOblot, it is probably easily reversable without chemo, radiation, or surgery. It's sad that most insurers won't pay for it.

pH Balance

Periodically, check your pH levels with a saliva test. Lump tumors are acidic, and bombarding them with alkalinity is a heavy weapon. Additionally, some blood cancers and lymphomas are alkaline.

So, a good pH balance is important. Acidity is a catalyst for disease. As a rule, cancer patients have a much higher acidity than normal. Some estimates are hundreds of times more acidic than those without the presence of cancer in the body. On the other side of the coin, people with normal blood chemistry have had high levels of acidity, and children with cancer have had high alkaline levels. But that's not what this is about. This is about general rules of thumb.

> *Whether you think you can or you think you can't, you're right.*
>
> —Henry Ford

There's No Money in Cures

If you cure a disease, you get paid once. If you find a drug to help the patient endure, you get paid indefinitely. You know the old cliché: give someone a fish or teach someone to fish. Cancer research is big business, and chemo drugs are one of the most profitable drugs ever produced. At the time of this writing, Jennifer has been a patient for about ten months. During that time, our cancer center and oncologist have billed our insurance company for hundreds of thousands of dollars.

That's a house with a pool. I'm not complaining about it because some of it worked, sort of. One of her tumors disappeared, and the other two were reduced in size by 25 percent, temporarily. Let's give credit where credit is due. This reduction in tumor size was due to a combination of radiation and immunotherapy. Unfortunately, it's a temporary fix. The downside is having some of your vital organs dissolved. Oh, well. In the meantime, the chemo continues to do what it always does best and disrupt the body's immune balance.

ENTER THE ONCOLOGIST

The oncologist is a physician who has received additional training to specialize in the treatment of cancer. Our oncologist was a nice enough chap, but when he walked into the room for our first meeting, I knew we weren't going to have a let's-get-to-know-each-other chat. He was much too important for that. We were not encouraged to ask questions, and there was no interaction at all between him and me.

Jennifer and I are of the generation where people wor-shipped their physician, who was the smartest person they knew and was never wrong. Unfortunately, we are not in Oz and the Wizard doesn't provide us with a brain. Physicians, as a rule, are well-meaning and caring. However, it's important to understand that they don't always go home and do research on weekends instead of playing golf. They make mistakes, and they don't have all the answers. It takes work to find new ways to do things, and it's uncomfortable and takes determination, but so what. Aren't you worth it? So then, sometimes the best thing to do is for you to do the work and the research and find out what is truly best for you.

Physicians want the best for their patients, but they have been discouraged from looking outside the box. Most will never cohabitate with integration because, apparently, medical schools do not waste their time with alternatives. The students are trained to cure with chemicals that, coincidently, are provided by the nice people who spend billions on medical schools and education. They basically go by the course prescribed by the name on the top left corner of the checks.

> *Security is mostly a superstition. Life is either a daring adventure, or nothing at all.*
>
> —Helen Keller

THE PHYSICIAN'S ASSISTANT

Our PA was one of the few people who appeared to care about us, as long as it didn't take up too much time. Our visits were designed for updates and med changes. In fact, the rare opportunity we had to ask health questions was with a PA. The PA is usually a very capable layperson who has been trained in the medical arts to relieve the workload of the physician for those areas that don't require the expertise of the big guy. Our PA was sympathetic and did everything allowable to help, but was obviously a product of the system. Apparently, our PA was kept on a fairly short lead totally within the box. It was another step in the process of dispensing drugs, crayons, and coloring books and stuff.

SUPPORT STAFF

Since no one can go directly to the PA or the Big Guy without first becoming a platinum club member, all clinical issues are referred in a strict chain of command that begins with the nice people behind the glass windows that separate them from reality. From there, it goes to the oncology nurse. Ours was never really much help, but always made up for it by being difficult to reach. We never felt like we got a thought past the dial tone.

THE COCKTAILS

In an NBC report by Rehema Ellis, Dr. Peter Einsberg states that oncology physicians are allowed to make a profit off of chemo drugs. This is not the case with traditional physicians and pharmaceuticals. Additional, Arthur Caplan, University of Pennsylvania Center for Bioethics, states that it is possible for a cancer physician to prescribe based on profit. This leaves the question, then: couldn't they prescribe for longer periods of time than necessary? Or couldn't they prescribe even when there is a question of its effectiveness, as in the case of my wife?

What would you do? It's no different than your auto mechanic selling you a fuel-injection system instead of telling you to change the type of fuel you are using. I said it before and will say it again, if they cure you, then you are off the payroll. There is no money in a cure. The smart money wants to keep you going. On two separate occasions, Jennifer had allergic reactions to the drugs. She had one to the immune stimulator that put her in the hospital for six days and one from the regular chemo that almost killed her while she was in the chemo chair. They had to call an ambulance to take her across the parking lot to intensive care. My belief, still, is that an RGCC Group test would have hinted that these particular chemicals may not be right. All that aside, I have to ask: if you are trying to stimulate the immune system, why not substitute the pembrolizumab with something like . . . say . . . vegetables? Is it just me?

> *Lean forward into your life. Begin each day as if it were on purpose.*
> —Mary Anne Radmacher

THE $64,000 QUESTION

If I said give me a quarter of a mil and I'll take it to

Vegas and put it on a number that has a 2.3 percent chance of winning, only unconscious people would agree to it. That's what Jennifer and I did. We paid over $300,000 to spin the wheel a few times. We tapped out.

So, why no diversity in medical school education? Much medical-school financing and research financing comes from people who have a vested interest in what they do with the money. Boards of directors of medical institutions have members who are directly connected to areas like pharmaceuticals and are discouraged from veering off course. It's kind of like eating your children.

Therefore, the trend toward natural medicine was squelched by 1950. Unless it's a secret, government intervention of monopolies has not reached the pharmaceutical industry. Disease has been defined as a marketplace, and it has been decided that an industry should be built upon it. Your local cancer center is, in fact, a business model. A very profitable one.

Think about it: every third advertisement on TV is selling drugs. Then, at the end, the happy couple is shown running down the beach laughing while the next sixty seconds or so are spent telling what could possibly happen to you with prolonged use. I guess if these people are laughing about it, how bad could it be? I'll take it.

A relative of mine wanted to take a medication to help alleviate acne. Then, the caregiver wanted to monitor liver function on a regular basis to make sure there was no loss of function. That's a fair trade. If someone threw a hundred-piece puzzle down on the table for you to put together, you would only need about half of the pieces in place before you knew what the picture was. If you see a barn, it's a safe bet there's a cow somewhere.

> *What am I living for and what am I dying for are the same question.*
>
> —Margaret Atwood

VARIOUS STUDIES

According to Mary Jo Parker, *How to Stop Your Metastasized Cancer*, university studies have shown that chemotherapy actually stimulates stem cells, and as a result, they come back even more aggressively and more malignant than when it started. The tumors are reduced in size because the chemo is reducing the size of the tumor cells, but not the stem cells. Here, again, the goal is a five-year success rate.

CHAPTER FOUR

WHO KNEW?

*When I hear people say, "Life is hard," I'm tempted
to ask, "Compared to what?"*

—Sydney Harris

WHY BOTHER WITH CONFLICTING DATA?

As I was gathering data, it started to look like the
private-sector data outweighed the data coming from the
National Cancer Institute or the American Cancer Society.
Others who have wondered the same thing say the cancer
giants fund primarily chemical cures. It makes sense that
they would not deviate from the bread and butter.

The more I thought about it, the more I realized there is
no incentive for the ACS or the NCI to do research
disputing the thousands of alternative researchers around
the globe. Why should they? It's not like they are going to
forego a trillion dollars in revenue to go home and do
blueberry smoothies.

If they found that there was a natural way, a better way,
to defeat cancer, would they use it? No, of course not. Let's

say the ACS really wanted to know if alfalfa juice squirted into your ear would cure a brain tumor. What if it worked? Then what? Since they can't patent it, how would they recover their investment? That's why they couldn't use Johanna Budwig's recipe. If I donate money or walk in your parade, it will help you find a cure, right? Unless you have been chained to a waterpipe in some basement for most of your life, you know that's a ridiculous thought. Put it out of your mind.

> *One day, the American Cancer Society will celebrate*
> *its three hundredth birthday.*
>
> —Frank Ruane

THE PET SCAN: CANCER'S LITTLE LOLLIPOP

PET stands for Positron Emission Tomography. Sounds innocent enough, but it's bad for you. It just happens to be the lesser of two evils. It's the Trojan horse approach. Tumors absorb sucrose many times faster than normal cells. They need a way to get radioactive dye to the tumors without showing up elsewhere in the film. So they take sucrose and impregnate it with the dye, inject it into the bloodstream, and voila! The tumors show up for a family photo. Some say it's a different type of sugar. Nope. Sucrose is the same and is metabolized the same on the molecular level.

THE REALITY OF A CURE

In 1908, one in thirty-three people would get cancer. In 2020, one in three will get cancer, and there has been no appreciable change in the cancer survival rate in fifty-five years. Allegedly, chemotherapy and mammography cause cancer, and modern medicine should know it. Those who have looked at the statistics will tell you that the cancer rate has increased 90 percent over the past fifty years. So, what's the deal with all the money that goes toward research and a cure?

Well, actually, that's it: follow the money. No one will ever walk into the oncology offices and labs and radiation facilities and send everyone home. It's just common sense, or, should I say, economics. We had muscular dystrophy telethons every August for forty-five years raising billions for research, and the average lifespan of a person with MD is still thirty years. From what I've read, only very few people live longer than that. Many believe the advances published are exaggerated. The hard reality is that cancer treatment hasn't advanced as much in fifty years as we would like to believe.

> *Every person who is alive today is someone who hasn't quit.*
>
> —Unknown

ANOTHER QUESTION YOU WANT THE ANSWER TO

Is the data from alternative medicine more reliable than

that of traditional medicine like the ACS and NCI? It takes a while to see what is happening. It's not necessarily more reliable, just different and, at times, more complete. The cancer establishments have a large, voracious appetite in their supporting companies to maintain. They have to keep others in the money loop, like people who make chemo paraphernalia and oncologists and drug companies and equipment for the chemo clinics, and it's an enormous empire with many mouths to feed. Doing trials on something that would produce no profit is bad business . . . allegedly. And it's understandable.

Additionally, natural cures can't be patented, because they are given by God or nature, depending on how you choose to believe. Therefore, a lot of time is spent just trying to prove alternatives wrong, going after the hole in the pocket. On the other side of the coin, however, is the research done by people who said there has to be a better way. One of the differences could be that many of these people haven't been on their knees asking God for a miracle for themselves or a loved one. In my opinion, one of the reasons alternative data is more reliable is because it comes from the heart and not the pocket.

THE NEED FOR MORE RELIABLE DIET INFORMATION

To reiterate, Jennifer and I had a ten-minute diet course, accompanied by some literature, while she was sitting in the chemo chair. Yep, it's an excellent time to be given a technical class. This was accompanied by an expensive-looking leather-bound diet portfolio. It was an impressive sight. However, it contained very little information that would truly help the body heal, and also some very bad suggestions for a cancer patient. I didn't realize how much they didn't tell us until I realized how much they didn't tell us.

It appeared as though the diet was designed to help the patient withstand chemo and not really to stop the growth of cancer in the body or even promote overall health, for that matter. There was no mention of things many consider important in curing cancer. I didn't want to put anyone on the spot, but I really wanted to know why.

Okay, so if there is really no cure, per se, what is going to happen? Well, I'm guessing the people in Vegas would say we will reach a point where you can live as long as you want (quality excluded) as long as you stay on the pre-scribed medication. That way everyone wins. You get to live to be ninety-five, and the pharmaceuticals make the big bucks while you do it. Everyone's happy. Sort of.

> *I have never in my life learned anything from any man who agreed with me.*
>
> —Dudley Malone

IS EARLY CANCER DETECTION A SCAM?

The science supports the theory of John McDougall, MD. According to Dr. McDougall, researcher, lecturer, and best-selling author, preventing cancer is the only positive solution. Early detection is not all it's cracked up to be, and it doesn't save the lives it has been credited for saving. For example, the breasts and the prostate each contain about one hundred billion cells. When a cell goes wild and becomes a cancer, it enters the doubling rate for cells, which is every hundred days. First one cancer cell, then in a hundred days, two cancer cells, then four and so on. Every doctor knows this. Therefore, at the end of about six years, the tumor is about the size of a pencil tip. Then, after about ten years, the tumor is about one centimeter, or the size of a pencil eraser.

This is when the tumor in the breast can be felt or the PSA in the prostate goes up. The medical course of action is to rush you into surgery, chemo, and radiation for something that has been growing for six, eight, or ten years. Maybe longer. It's not complicated. It's just math, and it is based upon science. They don't give you a chance to plan a course of action from sound advice and let you react out of fear and ignorance.

WHAT'S THE REAL DANGER?

Early detection isn't working. Sure, there are exceptions, and sure, there are remissions, but that's not the rule. I'm sorry. So where is the danger in misinformation? The real danger is that the language of the medical profession is often ambiguous. For example, when they find a tumor in more than one location, they say it has metastasized. Conversely, when they don't find any more tumors, they say it has not metastasized. Seems simple enough.

Here is where the danger begins: a tumor that is barely visible to the naked eye has, technically, already metastasized; it just hasn't gotten big enough to see in other areas yet. This is what happens in the magic kingdom of remission. Some treatment has shrunk a tumor, or tumors, but the circulating cancer cells or CTCs are present throughout the body and can surface anywhere. This characteristic is what makes strengthening the immune system so important. The body is the only thing that can heal on the quantum, or cellular, level.

THERE'S LOGIC IN NOT GETTING COLONOSCOPIES AND MAMMOGRAMS

Sound ridiculous? According to many experts, this is the advice of the Canadian Task Force on Preventive Health Care. They have finally realized that if you detect it with a colonoscopy, it is already a decade old, and colonoscopies are physically dangerous. Additionally, colonoscopies are expensive and a one-in-two-thousand chance you will suffer a perforation of the intestine. According to Dr. John McDougall, there is no evidence that colonoscopies save lives. A better approach is a two-foot-long tube inserted just to the colon. They call it endoscopy.

Lastly, mammograms probably give women breast cancer. It's not uncommon to have a mammogram and develop a tumor six months later. Most of the readers of this book have heard of a woman who has found a pencil eraser–sized tumor in a breast. By scientific math of calculating the doubling time of cancer cells, the tumor is ten to twelve years old. Then she gets a mammogram, and six months later the tumor is the size of a golf ball. Is it coincidence?

SHOULD MEN STOP HAVING THE PROSTATE CUT OUT?

Prostate cancer is one of the slowest growing of all. If you are over sixty and you have a positive PSA, you may not have a tumor but just cancerous cells. If, for example, you have two million cancer cells in the prostate, it may have taken years to get to that point. That's about the size of a pin head. We will most likely die of something else before the prostate tumor kills us. Here, again, before you bounce into the chemo ward or jump up on the table, take the time to do your homework.

When one door closes, another one opens. Or you can open the closed door. That's how doors work.

—Unknown

CHANCES OF SURVIVAL

Ivelisse Page was thirty-seven years old when she was diagnosed with Stage IIIA colon cancer. After further tests, it was discovered she had Stage IV cancer because it had spread to her liver. She refused chemotherapy and worked with a combination of a naturopathic physicians and oncologists from Johns Hopkins and used mistletoe therapy to cure her cancer. Mistletoe therapy is common in Europe. What is interesting, however, is when she asked her oncologist what her survival chances were with chemo and with doing nothing, his answer was 67 percent with chemo and 57 percent with just some minimal lifestyle changes. In many instances, the differences are only 2 percent. Let's be realistic. I'd take the 67 over the 57, but that's a neon sign flashing that says there are other options. With some thought, 10 percent shouldn't be so hard to make up, right? Right.

> *I am thankful for all of those who said no to me. It's*
> *because of them I'm doing it myself.*
>
> —Albert Einstein

IMMUNOTHERAPY

It was difficult writing this paragraph, because it hits so close to home. Recently, immunotherapy has become the little sister to chemo. As I mentioned earlier, Jennifer had considerable trouble with the immunotherapy that almost killed her and required six days of hospitalization and twenty-one days of steroids to restore her intestinal function.

Its claim to fame is that it encourages the immune system to attack invaders to the body. On the chalkboard, it seemed like a good idea. Unfortunately, as in the case of my wife, the chemicals are going to encourage the immune

system to go after anything, including normally function-
ing parts of the body. As I write this paragraph, Jennifer is
currently hospitalized in a struggle to rid her body of the
immunotherapy drugs. Basically, the cure is killing her.
Although she is gung-ho on traditional medicine, she had
debilitating colitis for two weeks. Incidentally, colitis is a
word they use when they don't know why your body is
draining itself of every ounce of fluid, and shredding its
organs, in an effort to survive. We had to rely on expensive
bags of chemicals to stop the ongoing diarrhea, and then
another three weeks of gradually diminishing steroids to
prevent it from reoccurring. What can I say?

Let me see if I have this straight. They gave her dangerous chemicals to help retard the cancer. She had a reaction
to them, and her body is fighting furiously to get rid of
them. So, they are giving her more dangerous chemicals to
stop her body from protecting itself against the dangerous
chemicals they gave her until she is well enough to take
another three-month round of dangerous chemicals.
Okay, sure, I can see the logic in that.

It's Not Just Cancer

Yes, this is primarily about the cancer-cure business.
However, it's important to understand that regardless of
the disease you are facing as a challenge, there are certain
consistencies that apply to it all. All disease is a breakdown of some part of the immune system.

- Drugs are the first thing thrown into the ring. Many have very low cure rates, and many have very dangerous side effects; some are lethal. Am I the only one who recognizes that every third advertisement is prescription drugs?

- The philosophy to understand here is that it's more than just eating raw fruits and vegetables and taking a few supplements. There is something else you are doing or eating that is causing the breakdown in your body's ability to manage itself. Strip down naked (chemically speaking) and start from scratch. Cleanse the body of all toxins and foreign substances, especially drugs, and do what needs to be done. Give your body a fighting chance.

Get busy living or get busy dying.
— Stephen King, *The Shawshank Redemption*

EDUCATION, NOT MEDICATION

I have not spent a lot of time answering specific questions, but rather have tried to open a realm of encouragement and an avenue to a new understanding. There are numerous websites, periodicals, and books to help you through your journey. One of these is the Truth About Cancer Ultimate Live Symposium. None of us are the same and not all cancers are the same, so venues like this are valuable because of the diversity they offer in the numerous treatment styles and opinions. The websites I reference are outstanding resources for information. Use them.

CHAPTER FIVE

MANY OTHERS HAVE BEEN SUCCESSFUL

Never look back unless you are planning to go that way.

—Henry David Thoreau

DIENEKE FERGUSON

Reportedly, in Britain, Dieneke Ferguson was diagnosed with a rare blood disease called multiple myeloma. She underwent three rounds of chemo and four stem-cell transplants, and nothing worked. This blood disorder is one where the white blood cells, which normally protect us from viruses, go wild and wreak havoc on the bones. She was told to get her affairs in order when she decided to take her health in her own hands. She took eight grams (two teaspoons) of curcumin daily for five years and completely eliminated her disease. Healthcare professionals at Baylor University as well as from prestigious London hospitals weighed in on her success and have agreed the radical transformation could only have come from her dietary and lifestyle changes. Unfortunately, until you can stuff a human into a flask, the research data is skewed.

STANISLAW BURZYNSKI, MD, PHD

Dr. Burzynski has impeccable medical credentials and operates a clinic in Texas where he has, for the last forty years, had success with a treatment called antineoplaston therapy. He is not only a medical doctor and oncologist, but has a PhD in biochemistry. His clinic has, reportedly, had success with rare forms of childhood brain cancers and such. There is too much conflicting data and too much medical and chemical jargon to list here. So, let's cut through the layers of jargon and look at one final logical point. The medical board of Texas and several other "prestigious" medical institutions have spent millions over the past forty years suing Dr. Burzynski and attempting to stop his practice. So, right now, ask yourself if they would go to all this trouble over someone who was really a quack. Read what you can about Dr. Burzynski's work and form your own conclusion.

WHAT ELSE IS IGNORED?

An early advocate of sugar-free cancer treatment is Johanna Budwig, MD, PhD. Dr. Budwig was a physician, held a PhD in biochemistry, and was trained in physics. Additionally, she was nominated for the Nobel Prize in medicine seven times. She is responsible for curing hundreds of cancer patients over a five-decade period until her death in 2003 at the age of ninety-five. In fact, she is credited with a 90 percent cure rate that included her Budwig Diet, which included her cottage cheese/flaxseed oil mix and refraining from sugar, meat, and any animal or trans fats.

Dr. Budwig took two primary ingredients and basically found a cure for cancer before the government shut her down. Dr. Budwig cured over 90 percent of her patients. Let me put that into perspective for you. If you have a 3 percent success rate with your research, you can get grants to continue. Of course, we pay for it, but who's counting? If you have a 3–5 percent success rate, you get mentioned in some publication. At 51 percent, you have a cure. Not a bad gig. It's like being able to give yourself pay raises. Sound familiar?

According to Kelly Turner, PhD, for every self-cure that is investigated by modern medicine, there are a hundred that are not. They call it spontaneous remission and say they don't know how it happens. There are no personal stories, no faces, just statistics. In her interviews with self-cure patients, she was told they were never asked how they did it by the medical community.

The Budwig Diet is recognized by open-minded physicians and researchers throughout the world. Dr. Budwig took simple ingredients and created a cure for cancer. That's what they say. This simple cure, supported by a diet of organic raw fruits and vegetables, was the diet shot heard around the world. Let me quote Dr. Budwig: "The

American doctors come here and see my work and are impressed. They want to make a special deal and take it back and make a lot of money off of it. I won't do it, so they blackballed me in every country." This leads us to the most common question of all: if it works, why don't we use it?

The answer is actually quite simple. The drug companies are not willing to invest in treatments that they can't patent. Why would they want to invest in a cure where they could not recover the investment for trials and study? You can't blame them. The catch-22, though, is that it leaves little light at the end of the tunnel to find a cure. T. Colin Campbell, in his book *The China Study*, agrees with Dr. Budwig on animal fat and points out that most of it is laced with hormones. My personal, uneducated opinion is that it is food with growth hormones that causes breast and prostate cancer. Then again, I just bounced off the turnip truck.

RESPONSIBLE PROFESSIONALS AROUND THE WORLD RECOGNIZED HER WORK

In the *Townsend Letter to Doctors*, July 1990, they stated, **"Dr. Budwig has shown us that curing cancer is relatively easy. The response is immediate and cancer cells are weak and vulnerable."** Speaking on behalf of Dr. Budwig, Dan Roeham, MD, FACP, said, "Even failed operations and x-ray therapy can be treated in a few months, I would say, 90 percent of the time. To my knowledge, it has not been contradicted, but this information has taken a long time to reach this side of the ocean, hasn't it. Cancer treatment can be very simple and very manageable if you know how. The cancer interests don't want you to know this. Forgive the miscreants who have kept this simple information from reaching you for so long."

THERE IS NO MAGIC BULLET; IT'S A MAGIC OVERHAUL

We have to get out of the magic bullet mindset. There is one thing that self-cures have in common; that is, they all did a radical diet change. They didn't just start taking extra herbs and supplements, but rather changed everything.

They stopped the intake of sugar, trans fats, meat, dairy, and the harmful substances. They replaced damaging diets with fresh, organic fruits and vegetables, juicing many times each day, purified water, immune-enhancing supplements, reducing stress, and attitude changes. So, it was an entire life change. They realized the cancer came from a lifestyle that was harmful and damaging to their overall health. Additionally, they all relied on intuition and instinct to find direction.

> *Darkness is needed to see the stars.*
> —Unknown

THE ROAD MOST TRAVELED

According to oncology nurse Valerie Warwick, "Oncologists are stretching the truth about cancer treatments."

Oncologists are encouraged to follow the standards for care set up by the National Comprehensive Cancer Network (NCCN) regardless of whether the treatment will work for the individual being treated. No two persons are exactly alike or respond the same to a given treatment. This is why sensitivity testing is important in selecting a course of treatment. It is now possible to narrow down the biochemistry of the individual to a particular type of cancer cell. This gives a specific definition of the cancer and gives valuable information on what it will respond to. The human body can be nourished into healing itself.

PROFESSIONALS RECOGNIZING THE PROBLEM

I have a client who works at a nearby car dealership who has told me on more than one occasion he would not bring his car there to be worked on or serviced. It's that way with many healthcare professionals. If it hasn't happened already, sooner or later they will be on the other side of the counter, and I can promise you it will be a game changer. It's different when it's you. So, would you still be willing to be serviced there, knowing what you know about it? I mentioned Valerie Warwick. She was an oncology nurse for seventeen years and gave up a good job because she was tired of what's being done in mainstream cancer treatment. And Ms. Warwick is one of many such courageous professionals.

WHAT ELSE CAN WE DO?

I've rambled on for several pages, and there is actually a reason for it all besides passing on information. So, what do we do with all this alternative information? Well, we had to put warnings on cigarette packs, and we had to start telling the truth on food packages. Restaurants have to tell you if there is gluten in any of their dishes, self-help books have a disclaimer, and we can find a history of repairs on a prospective vehicle purchase.

More than any country in the world, Americans rely on having a choice with everything. We now require truth in labeling on food products. Wouldn't it be a good idea to have a standard diet protocol that every cancer patient has access to, one that is not subject to the watchful eye of cancer interests and pharmaceuticals? Wouldn't it be a good idea if the cancer interests had to tell patients that there are other things that work as well that are a fraction of the cost? Then again, maybe carrots would go up to ninety-four dollars a pound. Jennifer was given a cancer diet that the government wouldn't allow in schools. Go figure.

> *The definition of insanity is doing the same thing repeatedly and expecting a different result.*
>
> —Unknown

THE BATTLE FOR DISCLOSURE AND TRANSPARENCY

We demand it in politics, why not here? I believe there

61

is enough scientific data and medical evidence to support changing the dietary criteria for cancer patients. I believe it reasonable and prudent to give the cancer patient all available information on other nutrition and treatment paths that would facilitate healing. We need a more pro-active approach that provides a "truth in advertising" at-titude, which allows patients to make intelligent, respon-sible choices in their healing process in spite of what the ACS objects to. Currently, this is not the case.

We, Jennifer and I, worked with one of the many prestigious cancer institutions in North Georgia. They are easier to find than donut shops. Cancer treatment is a very profitable business, and it's self-perpetuating. You can't ask for more than that. Much dietary literature, given to us by our dietitian, conflicts with data presented by brilliant scientists in every developed nation in the world. Hmmm. There's a dilemma.

LET'S TAKE A PEEK THROUGH THE ACS WINDOW

The ACS boasts a 2.3 percent total cure rate overall. It's about the same as it was in 1955. However, it's encourag-ing to think it could be up to 10 percent in, say, a genera-tion or so. Before you roll your eyes, remember that any recurrence of the cancer after five years doesn't count. If you make it five years and one hour, you win. You're in the cured stats. You get confetti and balloons and drinks on the house and stuff.

In recent years, the cost of drugs to treat cancer have

increased 5,000 percent. Also, the ACS is, allegedly, publicly committed to destroying every natural, nontoxic, cheap cure for cancer that exists and, allegedly, has business ties to organizations that develop chemotherapy equipment, make vaccines, and sell chemotherapy drugs, just to name a few. Add it all up and the ACS has an economy about the same as Brazil's.

Unless my information is incorrect, the board of directors of the American Cancer Society is comprised of five officers and sixteen members at large. The officers are medical professionals who would have some scientific knowledge of the cancer-healing process. Few have bios that would indicate anything outside the box of traditional medicine, which, as the world knows, is influenced by guess who. According to an uncategorized ACS post, one of the ACS board members is the CEO of a biotech company that sells chemotherapy equipment. What're the chances? Some other members at large are law, finance, and business oriented—the necessities for conducting Big Business. Seems reasonable.

An Example of Bureaucratic Wisdom (Yes, an Oxymoron)

I believe it helpful if we have some examples of what we are dealing with in Big Medicine, Big Business, or Big Government. Dr. Henry Heimlich was the developer of the Heimlich maneuver. In simplicity, this is a method of diaphragm compression that dislodges particles or water from the airway. Norman Vincent Peale is credited with saying that "Henry Heimlich saved more lives than any person in history."

According to reliable sources, the American Heart Association and the American Red Cross would not allow the maneuver to be used in any of their training programs. But wait, there's more! Instead, they advocated back-slapping, which lodges particles even deeper. It wasn't until Surgeon General C. Everett Koop told them to stop being stupid and get with the program that they reluctantly backed off.

> *You pray for rain, you gotta deal with the mud too.*
> *That's a part of it.*
>
> —Denzel Washington

WHAT ARE THE CHANCES OF UNBIASED RESEARCH?

The ACS is one of the largest contributors to cancer research. It looked mind-boggling to see the arenas they joust in, so we should break it down logically. Because of the huge money interest and ties with other businesses, it is illogical to assume the ACS looks at the benefits of alternative treatments. Why would it? Additionally, if they found a good alternative treatment, would they use it? Well, it depends on the money, which is the primary reason to spend more money to debunk alternative resources.

MEDICAL SCHOOLS HAVE THEIR HANDS TIED

Most of my source materials state that medical schools do not teach diet in the form of healing or preventive medicine. Medical school curriculums are chemical based, i.e. healing comes from drugs. Additionally, medical schools do not teach integrative approaches to medicine, especially cancer. The narrow scope of prescribed treatment is (a) surgery, (b) radiation, (c) chemotherapy. The truth is that physicians who deviate from this protocol risk losing their license. This comes straight from the horse's mouth (I think that's the part of the horse it comes from).

> *I've failed over and over and over again in my life,*
> *and that is why I succeed.*
> —Michael Jordan

THEIR CURIOSITY IS AROUSED

A team of American physicians, in the late 1980s, went to Germany and were impressed with the work Dr. Johanna Budwig was doing. They came back empty-handed when they realized they couldn't patent her cure or make any money off of it. According to Dr. Budwig's own words, she was, as I said earlier, blackballed. So where have they put us in the advancement arena? Well, under the watchful eye of the ACS, childhood cancers have increased 57 percent, and other cancers have increased as much as 168 percent, because we refuse to regulate the carcinogens being put into our food and our water.

Apparently, under the leadership and guidance of the ACS and NCI, several industries are linked together: pharmaceuticals, drugs, cosmetics, vaccines, drug-administering equipment, and others. What happened to the "monopoly" rule? I guess this is where we get the term "immune system." I know prescription drug abuse happens firsthand because it happened to Jennifer. She was taking nine of them. How does the human body process all this chemical information?

It's everywhere. Nutrition and the human body cure cancer. Many dietary restrictions stop the growth of tumors, but chemotherapy does not. The ACS should know it, the NCI should know it, the oncologists should know it, dietitians should know it, and physicians should know it.

ENTER OTTO WARBURG

Otto Warburg won the Nobel Prize in medicine in 1931 for his work on cell regeneration and glycolysis. This is a cell's demand for sucrose. Warburg discovered that cancer cells mainly rely on the first part of the energy-production process, which is dependent on glucose (sugar).

He noted that cells rely on glycolysis even if oxygen is present. Basically, Dr. Warburg found that cancer cells use oxygen differently than normal cells, called anaerobic glycolysis. The difference is in the kind of respiration the cells do. Dr. Warburg was able to turn a normal cell into a cancer cell just by depriving it of oxygen. How, then, do we deprive normal cells of oxygen? One very important way is diet. Where have we heard that before?

Then, the cancerous cells are dependent upon fermentation to survive. An interesting point is that, except for Jennifer's dietitian, the vast majority of cancer researchers agree with this.

Warburg is one of a long line of scientists, researchers, biochemists, physicians, and oncologists who have been fighting the trends of traditional medicine. These people understand the financial implications of deviating from the prescribed course of treatment.

I mentioned earlier that chemotherapy does not kill circulating tumor cells or stem cells. One of the other drawbacks to this is that these CTCs can still be enhanced by glycolysis or the absorbing of sucrose for energy. Research is showing that the ketogenic diet is the way to starve the cancer cell of oxygen without cutting off the supply to healthy cells.

IT'S MORE THAN JUST THE SUGAR

Although it's accepted that cancer cells absorb sugar eighteen times faster than normal cells, don't let that oversimplify the Warburg discovery. One of the glitches is that all cells use sugar, but to varying degrees. Dr. Warburg's work has been studied a lot in recent years, and it is important to understand that cancer cells don't need oxygen to process the sugar the way normal cells do.

CHAPTER SIX

A GUIDE TO WHAT WORKS

The difference between genius and stupidity is that genius has its limits.

—Albert Einstein

THE LOGICAL QUESTION IS, WHAT HAS WORKED FOR OTHERS?

As a rule, no one quits a job until they have another one. The first word that has to be included in what works is commitment. If you are going to walk away from Big Medicine chemo, you need to have an alternate plan and vow to be committed to it.

You must be committed to ninety days of total, radical life change with an understanding of what you can, and can't, do, eat, or drink. You can't look back. You can't waver in your decision. A chain is only as strong as the weakest link. You can't just walk away from Big Business medicine with nowhere to go. You must have a plan and be prepared to stick to it.

IT HAS TO BE MORE RADICAL THAN THE CANCER

When you walked into the Big Business cancer office, you walked into a painful climb to an obscure possibility of total success. When you make the decision to enhance traditional medicine with alternatives, you have made the decision to take control of your own life. It will most likely be the first, and last, life-and-death struggle you will ever have. It has to be a 100 percent commitment to healing with a total reversal of your old lifestyle. Ask for the encouragement of family and friends, and don't let discouragement sway you. They have the same conditioning you are fighting right now. Draw a line in the sand.

FASTING

Fasting is one of the oldest mechanisms for healing since man first walked the planet. Biblically, it was expected you would fast, and it was common to fast one full twenty-four-hour day per week. It doesn't say if you fast, it says *when* you fast. A fast, however, is a radical treatment, and seriously ill people should consult their caregiver before starting one. Healthy people, however, should make it a regular part of their diet. There are numerous good books on the benefits of fasting for you to research. Do it now. Don't wait.

ESSIAC TEA

Essiac tea comes from the great northland of Canada. A nurse by the name of Rene Caisse (Essiac spelled backward) is credited for bringing it to the attention of the people of North America after a chance encounter who had been cured of cancer by it. The concoction was formulated by a member of the Ojibwa tribe in Canada, where a medicine man gave it to an English tradesman to cure him of cancer. Rene used it successfully in the early part of the twentieth century. Nurse Caisse treated thousands of cancer patients successfully beginning in 1922. She took no money and had a letter sent on her behalf by eight physicians to the Canadian Health Authority. As in the United States, she would have been arrested, except for the fact that she had accredited physicians backing her. The cancer interests will not allow an herbal cure. Period.

It would not only be well worth your while to read her story, but you will find it very encouraging as well. The exact formula has been passed down, and you will have to do some research to find the correct one. However, I would not use tablets or a powder, as the herbs have to be boiled and brewed for ten to twelve hours and must contain the root of sheep sorrel. It has been said that there is no evidence of her cures, but this is not true, as she used the formula successfully from 1922 until her death in 1978 at the age of ninety-one.

DON'T UNDERESTIMATE

You may be thinking that alternative cures are rare and randomly selected. Actually, the reverse is true. Nutritional cures have a high success rate, whereas Big Cancer still falls into the low-percentage category for a complete cure. Yes, I remember, there are a lot of different kinds of cancer.

COFFEE ENEMAS

At the last minute, I decided to add this, because people have been asking me if I've heard of this treatment and if it works. Well, yes, I have, and I don't know if it works. They have been around for a long time. Proponents say they stimulate enzymes in the liver that have a cleansing effect on the body overall. The data is ambiguous. Hollywood notables have tried them over the years, but I have been unable to find any evidence that they work. Like everything else, someone had to try it the first time for some reason. It was probably at a frat party, but your guess is as good as mine. Do your homework.

LOW-DOSE NALTREXONE

Naltrexone is a nontoxic drug that has shown great promise in reducing tumors and combating the HIV virus, as well as certain types of melanomas. It goes against all prescribed cancer treatments because it's inexpensive. How can that happen? To find out how Naltrexone works, go to the website of David Gluck, MD, at www.ldninfo.org. Here you will find information on treatments for about 450 people that were, statistically, very successful.

LIQUID NUTRITION

In addition to any protocol you choose, you will be most likely drinking eight or more glasses of raw, organic fruit and vegetable juices. Purchase a good juicer that is up to the task of the daily use it will be getting for the next ninety days.

Select the store where you will purchase your fruits and vegetables. Don't be afraid to try new things. Read the diets others have used successfully and imitate them. Also, this is not a time when you need negativity in your life. Keep only positive, supportive people around you. Stay away from those who disagree with you or bring doubt into your life.

HYPERTHERMIA

I was interviewed by an author while traveling on a train several years ago. It's easy to get into conversations on trains because you are basically locked in. She was doing research because a clinic in Canada was having great success with hyperthermia and cancer, and it was suddenly closed. She was interested in what I had to say because I personally knew two people who were going to die from cancer, came down with a fever for no reason, and then the cancer was gone.

The data suggests that it is a good practice to get into a sauna to raise the body's temperature five or six degrees for short periods of time to help destroy disease. This is one of the few areas where reading about it is not boring and technical, but rather quite interesting.

PROTOCEL

Protocel is a very interesting but very touchy subject. It has been around for a few decades now and has many, many documented cases of cures for several different types of cancer, but Big Money cancer hates it. To keep Big Business from scratching your eyes out, it can only be advertised as a dietary supplement. Protocel was previously marketed as Cancell by Jim Sheridan and has a very specific protocol for taking the formula. The administration of the drug was detailed very nicely in the book *Outsmart Your Cancer* by Tanya Harter Pierce, and it is one of the more encouraging compounds to come along.

The really good news is that the Food and Drug Administration and National Cancer Institute have both condemned it vigorously. They more they protest, the more likely it is to be a good product. They don't bother with all-out campaigns against supplements that are not promising. It appears that any attempt at stopping the goose that lays the golden pills is squelched.

Additional Thoughts

- Stay positive. Attitude is everything. Most of all, don't let them rush you into anything. Time is on your side, not against you.

- Clean up your environment. Stop all chemicals like cleaning fluids, makeup, and foods with additives and such.

- Stop eating harmful food products like sugar, meat, trans fats, dairy, and nonorganic. Note: Regardless of how much other research is out there, there is enough conclusive evidence to make it worthwhile to stop these harmful foods and additives. The very worst thing it can do is help.

- Look into the miracle herbs: curcumin, high doses of turmeric, black cumin seed oil, vitamin D, vitamin B12, sunshine, vitamin C, juicing, and organic vegetables and fruits and a lot of them. Frankincense oil has been used to cure many ailments and was given to the Christ Child. Many believe the gold was not the metal but actually turmeric, since the other two gifts were medicines also. Essential oils are just that, essential.

- BEC5 sometimes can be purchased and has been shown to cure skin cancer. It comes from the devil's apple plant in Australia and was first used by Dr. William Chan. It cures by attaching itself to the sugar receptors, and the cancer cells basically digest themselves to death. It was sold over the counter and cured seventy thousand cases of skin cancer until, unfortunately, the Australian dermatologists complained and said it had to be prescribed by a physician.

- Manage your stress. Look at the word: dis-ease.

- Rely on your instincts and intuition. People who were interviewed about how they healed themselves all said they knew how they got sick and instinctively knew what needed change. It's true. You know about the cheeseburgers you've eaten and the desserts and soft drinks and pizza and not eating enough fruit and veggies. It's not a secret, and it's not a surprise to you. Change.

- Drink only high-pH purified water. Acidic bodies are sick; alkaline bodies are healthy. Track your progress or have your healthcare professional track it for you. Even better. It will give you concrete evidence of a cure.

- Read everything constructive that you can to learn how to manage your health and stimulate your immune system. After all, that's what this is all about—stimulating your immune system enough to heal you completely.

DETOXIFICATION

To get a jump start on your healing process, it helps to detox your body. There are numerous ways to do this. You can drink a lot of water, which you should be doing anyway, and eat the foods that help move toxins through your body quickest and most efficiently. One of the best foods you can eat for this is organic broccoli sprouts. Broccoli sprouts have the highest concentration of sulforaphane, which helps your liver clean itself. It's extremely powerful.

When your car is stuck on the railroad tracks, indecision is a decision.

—Unknown

THE BUDWIG PROTOCOL (THE SIMPLEST CURE OF ALL)

1. In a bowl, put six tablespoons of organic cottage cheese or quark.
2. Add three tablespoons of cold flaxseed oil (Barlean's is good).
3. Blend at slow speed for one minute with an immersion blender.
4. Add one teaspoon of raw organic honey.
5. Grind two tablespoons of raw organic flax-seeds. Use within fifteen minutes, because the seeds will lose potency after that.
6. Add to the bowl and mix.

7. Add organic fruit or turmeric, if desired, and serve in a small glass/porcelain container. Take twice daily, once in the morning and once in the evening. Don't take any other supplements except for the possibility of Poly-MVA

8. You should be taking two tablespoons of black cumin seed oil daily. Once in the morning and once at night.

9. Juicing is mandatory. Eight glasses of raw, organic vegetable juices should be ingested throughout the day.

10. Also, with any cancer diet, you will be eliminating anything that comes from an animal. Look at the diet recommendations of those who have been successful, like Chris Wark, Carla Camarillo, Kris Carr, April Saul, Dr. John Kelly, and others. Watch the interviews for the inspiration and the knowledge to know there is a lot out there that you can do that totally cures without destroying your immune system.

BUDWIG PROTOCOL?
SOMETHING SO SIMPLE. WHAT'S ALL THE FUSS?

Johanna Budwig's work was primarily related to the study of essential fatty acids and the importance of getting them back into our diets on a regular basis. Dr. Budwig also found that the body assimilated EFAs more efficiently when combined with sulphur-based proteins such as those found in yogurt and cottage cheese. This, in combination with foods rich in essential fatty acids like flaxseed oil, had amazing healing effects on the body. Nature actually combines these two for us in several foods like nuts and milk.

> *Don't cry because it's over. Smile because it happened.*
>
> —Unknown

FILTER YOUR WATER

Our drinking water contains harmful chemicals, intentionally put in there, that will hurt your recovery chances. Some of these chemicals are chlorine and fluoride, and they should be filtered out before drinking. Fluoride is one of the worst chemicals we consume on a regular base and has been linked to bladder cancer, lung cancer, liver cancer, cancers of the mouth and throat, and good grief. It is also present in diet sodas, beer, wine, and some juices. There are excellent filters out there, but make sure it is one that double filters and removes these harmful chemicals as well as bacteria- and water-borne diseases. If you can think about it for short bursts so you don't get too depressed, cancer is a self-perpetuating industry. It's like being forced to buy gasoline that's bad for your engine. We have choices, of course, but they're all different degrees of bad. Good work if you can get it.

Avoid Toxic Metals

This is a complex area, and I promised I would keep the technical data to a minimum. The simplest thing to do is avoid all animal foods, meat and dairy, as they are loaded with contaminating metals like mercury. Read the reports on ingredients. Fortunately, toxic metals can be eliminated from your body in about four months, but you have to stop putting more back in.

A Thought for the Good People Who Gave My Wife Her Institutional Cancer Diet

There are some worthwhile suggestions in the diet. Thank you for that. The glitch is that they won't override what it lacks or the harm it potentially could do. When I started having some questions about the entire process, I had already heard about sugar and the debate over giving it to cancer patients. I spoke with a pleasant young dietitian about the prescribed diet and asked why they allowed all the junk food and sugar. Our dietitian said the need to avoid those foods is just a myth found on the internet.

Okay, first of all, the internet is just a vehicle that can carry you anywhere around the world. It doesn't have an opinion. It doesn't wake up one morning and decide to pick on you. Secondly, the Tooth Fairy is a myth. Here, there is too much quality science from brilliant people behind it, and "myth" is an unfair and inaccurate word to use. Please stop using it. Bless your heart.

The information advising against sugar-laden junk food has been formulated by some of the finest clinical minds available internationally. The information is prolific and worldwide. The only base discrepancy is whether a tumor responds the same way as an individual cell in the laboratory, and research has found it does not. Here is some information to think about:

- When the NCI and the ACS don't know, they frequently say "there is no supporting evidence" or "studies aren't conclusive." Well, yes there is, and yes they are. Also, many dietitians are part of the industrial cancer complex without even knowing it. Like physicians, they are not encouraged to think outside the box.

- Reportedly, sugar activates oncogenes in tumors. It has been proven in the laboratory by PhDs in regenerative biology. Also, the University of Southern California has shown how cancer cells use sugar to grow, and Hoffmann–La Roche used strict laboratory studies to show cancer cells use sugar to create a protective shield against their attackers like white blood cells. Lorenzo Cohen, PhD, says, "We have determined specifically how fructose in table sugar and high-fructose corn syrup, ubiquitous within our food system, are responsible for facilitating lung metastasis in breast tumors." In the cancer research world, this is big. Think, for a moment, about the implications of this finding.

- The dietary considerations we were given do not mention organics when speaking of fruits and vegetables. Cancer patients need for their immune systems to concentrate on removing cancer waste, not pesticides and growth hormones. You don't have to read between the lines.

- The prescribed diet, even if the foods were all correct, does not provide for additional antioxidants needed to offset the oxidation and free radical stress imposed on the body by chemo and radiation. The longest-living people on earth are also the least sickly. They eat diets that are 95 percent plant based. They don't send out for Chinese.

- It is common knowledge among researchers of developed nations that the hormones IGF-1 and methionine are necessary for cancer growth and are found in meats. The more methionine contained in the food, the more it encourages the growth in cancer cells.

- Fish eat smaller fish, which eat the chemical contaminants of the sea like tuna fish eat mercury. A person on an anti-cancer diet doesn't need the extra pollutants, and they all need to be filtered from the body's bloodstream.

- Shellfish like oysters, crabs, lobster, and such should be avoided. Even the Bible says so. Also, fish off the coast of California have been found to contain radioactive materials from the three hundred tons of contaminated water that leaked out from the TEPCO power plant meltdown in Japan.

- Nearly 89 percent of the antibiotics sold in the US are used on animals that are being raised for food.

- Dairy products contain growth hormones that are designed to let a calf grow into a cow in six months. These hormones are not something a healing cancer patient should have.

- There are numerous herbs and spices that have been shown to stop the growth of tumors and even reverse them. Among these are amla, turmeric, curcumin, broccoli sprouts, and wheatgrass, to name a few.

- Also, cooking meat at high temperatures creates cancer-causing compounds called heterocyclic amines (HCA) and polycyclic aromatic hydrocarbons (PAH), which have been linked to colon, kidney, lung, and prostate cancer. People with the highest consumption of meat have a 70 percent greater risk of developing pancreatic cancer. Even the dead bacteria in meat causes inflammation in the intestines.

- Last but not least, survivors who are not in remission but have been totally cured are the true test. Those cured by alternatives outnumber those cured by chemotherapy, considerably.

POLY-MVA

Poly-MVA is one of the newer chemical compounds used in the fight against cancer. It can be purchased online and has had results in treating cancers of the lung, prostate, and breast by providing true alkalinity and antioxidants to the body. Reportedly, the effectiveness did not diminish with cancers that had metastasized. It can't hurt to check it out (James Forsythe, MD, HMD).

The best way out is always through.
—Robert Frost

USES FOR THE MICROWAVE OVEN

I can't think of any.

IS CANCER A FUNGUS?

I don't know, but there is encouraging research, to say

the least, that suggests bicarbonate solutions can be used to treat cancer the way it is used to treat fungi, as there are more than base similarities between the two. Dr. Tullio Simoncini is the Italian oncologist whose work is the foundation for the study that has shown that the alkaline bicarbonate solution injected into the tumor kills the tumor. Dr. Simoncini treats his patients for short periods of time, either in hospitals or having them stay at nearby hotels in Rome. While in medical school, Dr. Simoncini learned of the similarities between cancer and fungi and believed cancer would respond to therapies usually reserved for fungi. Reportedly, Dr. Simoncini's treatments have had amazing results. With camera views of the internal organs of cancer patients, Dr. Simoncini noted that the tumors were always white because of the fugal characteristics. According to the data I read, the tumors have diminished after his treatments—not in months, but in days.

KETOGENIC DIET DEBATE

The ketogenic diet is a high-fat, moderate-protein, no-carb diet. When you fast, the body goes into ketosis and switches from burning glucose for energy to burning fat. The reasoning is that cancer cells primarily feed on glucose and have a hard time converting fat to energy. Reportedly, the ketogenic diet starves cancer cells and they die. The fact is that cancer cells require eighteen times more sucrose (sugar) than normal cells, regardless of what the dietitian says.

On the theoretical basis, if you starve the cancer cells of

sugar by having a zero-sugar intake, the cells would die. On the practical side, however, too much of the body, like your brain, requires sucrose to survive. So, the solution is to force the body to start producing ketones. Then the brain, and other organs, can switch its metabolism over to burn the ketones instead. An ideal blood-sugar level would be about 60–80 mg/dl. Also, fortunately, cancer cells don't burn ketones.

Additional views on dietary considerations, like those from Mary Jo Parker, for example, include a ketogenic approach. Also suggested is antidiabetic medication, like Glucovance, to reduce the insulin levels in the blood, restricting protein intake, and the use of 2-Deoxy-D-glucose twice daily when blood sugar is at its lowest. This compound has been shown to inhibit the growth of tumors by stopping or greatly reducing the supply of glucose, the primary fuel for tumors. Do your homework on this and make decisions based upon the latest and most reliable information available. There's a lot of it.

COMPLEMENTARY ALTERNATIVE MEDICINE (CAM)

If there is anything that is becoming apparent, it's that there is a reason that many mainstream cancer interests are going to a combined or complementary method of treatment. When the smoke clears, you can see that traditional approaches aren't working and are bankrupting families with no results. The nontraditional approaches are holding up more than their end of the duo.

Complementary approaches are less radical than total lifestyle changes, and can dramatically reduce the effects of chemo and radiation. Additionally, they can help strengthen the immune system and reduce the effects of the poisons being introduced into the body. One of the major drawbacks against the CAM programs is that they are frequently administered by dietary professionals and not medical professionals and lose some credentials.

These are also called integrative therapies. Additionally, time should be allowed for them to start working on the system and should be followed for two weeks or more before starting chemotherapy. Don't count them out. Anything that enhances your chances of recovery is worth looking into.

THE ASPIRIN APPROACH

The drug question actually boils down to simplicity. When you take an aspirin for a headache, it doesn't cure the cause of the headache. The aspirin thins the blood so the problem doesn't affect us as much, and we get the illusion of pain relief. It's just that, an illusion.

If you had to take an aspirin every night to sleep through a headache, you would eventually have to get the cause of the headache fixed, or die. Cancer doesn't just happen for no reason. Fix the cause and stop fueling it.

Be all in or be all out, but choose.

—Unknown

What's the Bottom Line,
and What Am I Looking for?

Good question. Let's cut to the chase. I haven't been rambling just to see my words on paper. At this very minute, as I write these words, Jennifer is in the next room suffering like a goddamn lab rat, and it may have been preventable.

Here are my five goals:

First: If I can make one other person aware of the endless possibilities in alternative cancer cures and extend or save just one life, then my work will have been worth it.

Second: Cancer patients are entitled to have a choice and be given information on alternative and complementary solutions. It's an archaic concept called truth in advertising. Maybe you've heard of it. If Jennifer was given the same information from her oncologist that alternatives may have offered, she would have followed it unconditionally because of her trust in him. That's what I mean by conditioning.

Third: let's put pressure on the insurance companies to recognize viable alternatives and pay for them. The information is out there; let them look it up like you're doing. Reduce the pressure from Big Pharma.

Fourth: Let's find more healthcare professionals who recognize and prescribe out-of-system tests that could give life-saving information. I could be wrong, but I believe an RGCC group could have saved Jennifer from two lengthy stays in the hospital by giving us a hint on what her tumors would not respond to. Simple as that. The government calls it transparency, I think. You get it with your breakfast cereal, so why not here? It's common senses that has been smothered in billions of pharma dollars, and it needs to be exposed to save lives.

Fifth: Encourage healthcare professionals to provide a plan for eliminating or reducing long-term medications. Long-term meds are always harmful. Their benefits are limited, temporary, and most often the lesser of two evils.

If That's All There Is

If you are still thinking surgery, radiation, and chemo without looking elsewhere first, I don't know what more I can say. More than one source has said the average cancer patient is worth about $300,000 to the industry, and we passed that months ago. More families go bankrupt due to cancer treatment than any from other financial strain. So far, the miracles of modern medicine have allowed Jennifer to have a miserable, subhuman, barely tolerable existence for a whole year. A bargain at twice the price. It reminds me of the words to an old song by Peggy Lee, "Is That All There Is?" And she's right. If that's all there is, let's break out the booze and have a ball.

A Final Closing Thought

On February 27, 2019, Jennifer lost her battle with this disease. I believe she should still be here, and I believe she could have had two or three more comfortable years. There were several years of age between Jennifer and I, but she was my wife and the love of my life. To me, she's not just another statistic or another failed research blob, and I made a promise that I would do something useful with what I have learned through her ordeal.

The official cause of death is listed as "cardiac arrest and gram-negative septic shock." Is it blowing smoke? Based upon what I witnessed every day for thirteen months, my personal belief is that Jennifer did not die from cancer. I believe she died from drug overdose and immune system collapse. I watched it unfold firsthand over the months that she suffered. I will readily admit I have the bias of strong feelings involved in my belief. However, I saw the uncertainty, the ambivalence, and the trial and error. I watched firsthand the one-trick pony they call chemo. I sat with her in the middle of the night with my face pressed against hers while she cried. I held her while she vomited into a trash can and took drug after drug trying to find some relief. We have to stop the insanity. There has to be a better way.

Last Christmas, we lost our dog Toby to kidney failure. It happens with big dogs. He was part of our family, and we miss him greatly. The good people at the veterinary clinic felt bad that they could not save him, and they sent us a sympathy card that many people signed. It meant a great deal to us, and I still have it. In retrospect, Jennifer was a patient at the same cancer center for well over a year. During this time, she worked closely with an oncologist, an oncology nurse, chemotherapy staff, and a physician's assistant. We got nothing—not a card, a phone call, an email, a social media blurb, or a homing pigeon with a note . . . nothing.

REFERENCES

Carl Helvie, RN, PhD – Nutritional expert and forty-year lung-cancer survivor

Chris Wark – Author of *Chris Beat Cancer*. As one who self-defeated cancer, Chris has had a profound impact on the way we look at a formerly dreaded disease.

D. James Morré, PhD – Dr. Morré, professor emeritus of chemistry at Purdue University, received his doctorate in biochemistry from the California Technical Institute and is currently CEO and director of the MorNuCo research facility in Indiana.

Dennis Burkitt, MD (1911–2003) – Surgeon, researcher, lecturer; also famous for his work on starches and fiber.

Dr. Robert Eslinger – Medical director, Reno Integrative Medical Center

Galina Migalko, MD – Physician and researcher who has gotten international recognition for her work in the early detection of cancer.

Irina Kossoviskaia, MD, PhD – Physician, scientist, lecturer, and SCENAR expert

Ivars Kalvins, PhD – Dr. Kalvins was a 2015 finalist in the European Awards in Medicine

James Forsythe, MD, HMD – Cancer Treatment Center of Nevada

Jane Mclelland – Cancer survivor and author of *How to Starve Cancer*

Johanna Budwig, MD (1908–2003), Founder of the Budwig Protocol – Dr. Budwig was a biochemist and researcher for more than sixty years and also held doctoral degrees in physics and chemistry. During this time, her work became world renowned by using omega-3 fatty acids as a basis for her research on curing cancer through diet. She is credited with curing 90 percent of the patients sent to her and was nominated for the Nobel Prize in medicine seven times.

John Kelly, MD – Author of *Stop Feeding Your Cancer*

John McDougall, MD – Dr. McDougall is not only a physician, but an author and motivational speaker, and has been lecturing on the benefits of diet and exercise for decades. He was one of the first medical professionals to publicly speak out about modern medical treatments.

Kelly Turner, PhD – Harvard University and PhD from USC. Author of *Radical Remission: Surviving Cancer against All Odds.*

Mary Jo Parker – Author of *How to Stop Your Metastasized Cancer* and dietary counselor, bachelor's in nutrition from Cornell University, master's in clinical nutrition from State University of New York, professor of nutrition Canisius College

Patrick Quillin, MD – Former director of nutrition, Cancer Treatment Centers of America

Roby Mitchell, MD – Practices innovative and functional medicine in Amarillo, Texas

T. Colin Campbell, PhD – Author of *The China Study*

Tanya Harter Pierce, MA, MFCC – Author of *Outsmart Your Cancer*

The Truth about Cancer: A Global Quest – Nine-episode exposé on cancer treatment

Tullio Simoncini, MD – Oncologist responsible for research recognizing fungal properties of tumors

Valerie Warwick, RN – Valerie was an oncology nurse for seventeen years. After being discouraged by some of the practices of standardized medicine, she left the industry and spends her days lecturing, writing, and exposing the ineffectiveness of routine cancer therapy. Valerie tutors through her own website.

REFERENCE SITES

www.chrisbeatcancer.com – Chris Wark, author of *Chris Beat Cancer*, was diagnosed with colon cancer and chose to forego chemo and radiation and substitute nutrition for it. He cured himself and currently conducts regular interviews with many others who have done the same thing.

www.cancerwarrior.com – A group of women who have defeated breast cancer, and others, without chemo or radiation share their stories.

www.mywellnesstutor.com – Valerie Warwick was an oncology nurse before leaving the practice due to what she saw happening within cancer treatment. She spends her time now helping those who would like to know the truth about Big Business medicine.

www.beatcancer.org – The Center for Advancement in Cancer Education offers information, training, and seminars about cancer treatment without lethal drugs and radiation.

www.naturalnews.com/beatcancer – This site was founded by Mike Adams, the Health Ranger. Mike operates health spas and has written over two thousand articles on health maintenance through nutrition.

www.cancertreatments.net – A generic site that gives treatment information from both sides of the aisle.

www.drugdangerous.com – This is an informative site that offers information on the serious side effects of prescription drugs as well as recall information. It provides a good review of any medications you may be taking and offers questions to ask your doctor.

www.radicalremission.com – The site, and book, *Surviving Cancer against All Odds*, by Kelly Turner, PhD, offers a wide insight into the healing powers of whole foods.

www.greenmedinfo.com – This site looks at the fact that natural aids and remedies are not alternative, but have become alternative since science has taken over our healthcare.

www.annieappleseedproject.org – A project that was developed as a result of Ann Fonfa's desire to provide alternative health information. A breast cancer survivor since 1993, Ann's site has reached eight thousand pages.

www.cancercrackdown.com – A nonprofit organization that offers a wide variety of cancer options and treatments from the patient perspective.

Frank Ruane

www.atkins.com – This site deals with information on low-carb diets.

www.polymva.com – Poly-MVA is a supplement that is not only an antioxidant, but offers cell oxygenation and helps prevent cell damage from free radicals.

www.cancertutor.com – Takes an encompassing look at reducing toxicity in the body in an effort to help the body heal in an alkaline environment.

ABOUT THE AUTHOR

Frank Ruane is a native of Portland, Maine, but was raised in the Washington, DC, area. He worked there as an electrician and electrical contractor until moving to the Atlanta area with his wife and youngest son in 1998. Frank took an early retirement from the electrical industry in 2009 to pursue other interests and currently resides in their North Georgia home.